NOCTURNAL BREATHING IN AUTISM SPECTRUM CHILDREN:

COMPARATIVE EVALUATION OF MELATONIN AND MOZART EFFECTS

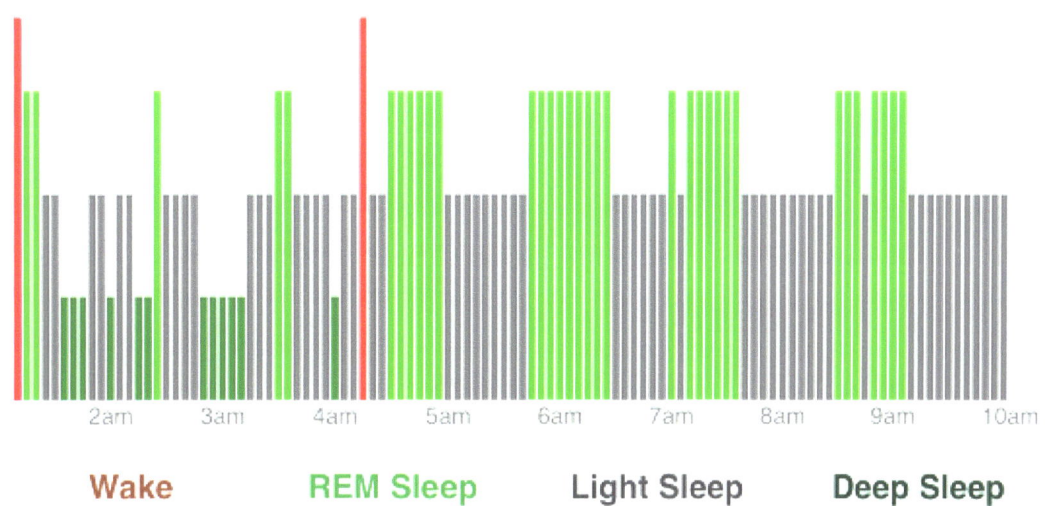

Dedicated to Mayo Clinic Foundation

by Naira R. Matevosyan, MD, PhD

Copyright © 2011 Naira Matevosyan, "L'auteur" librairie"

CreateSpace, Inc. ISBN: 978-1466438767; North Charleston, SC

CONTENTS:

ABSTRACT

OBJECTIVES: To determine: (1) the developmental phenotype and components associated with sleep disorders; (2) comparative sleep battery in children with autism spectrum syndromes; and (3) alternative practices in alleviating sleep symptomatic repeatedly reported in autism spectrum disorders (ASD).

METHODS: Of the total 148 retrieved papers, 64 studies of I-IIIA-level evidence pertaining to quantitative measures on development and sleep macro-structure from a sample of 1,823 ASD children and 1,190 typically developing peers (TDP), are allocated for the meta-assessment. Autism symptoms and sleep battery (total sleep time, sleep onset latency, REM latency, arousal index, periodic limb movement index, apnea, bruxism, sleep efficiency, other parasomnias) derived from subjective (provider and parental inventories) and objective measures (nocturnal polysomnography, actigraphy) are considered as measurable outcomes. Numerical outcomes encountered for ASD and hypnogrammes are assessed through the Pearson correlations.

RESULTS & CONCLUSIONS: Fairly different in expressions, prevalence of sleep onset disorders, sleep fragmentations, nocturnal breathing disorders, and reduced sleep efficiency are twice higher in children with Autism, Rett, Tourette`s, Angelman, and Heller`s syndromes. The age of Asperger`s children, does not relate to sleep problems other than central apnea (-0.8957) and daytime sleep duration (0.9226). Sleep symptomatic, especially parasomnias, are not related to children's cognitive and intellectual deficits, except of in Tourette`s children whose cognitive scores are negatively related to sleep onset parameters (- 0.9017). Sleep-maintenance insomnia and inefficient sleep have moderate associations with the central apnea, arousal index-having acceptable sensitivity (87%), and low specificity (26%). Exogenous melatonin improves sleep-wake cycles (60%), advances sleep-onset latency, however, does not impact on the arousal index. Findings inform the extensions of research in Mozart`s effect -as a natural stimulant of the endogenous melatonin.

KEYWORDS: Autism spectrum, sleep architecture, apnea, melatonin, Mozart effect

INTRODUCTION

Autism is one of the most prevalent global health problems with a ten-fold increase over the last decade. Yet, the totality of epidemiological evidence is not persuasive. The surveillance is affected with the fact that autism is often confused for its overlaps with other neuro-genetic syndromes, such as Angelman, Asperger`s, Heller`s, Lennox-Gastaut, Rett, or Tourette syndromes. Difficulties in definitions are derived of extreme paucity and complex interplay of autism spectrum disorders (ASD), hard to scale or judge with the help of the existing questionnaires.

The diagnostic inventories are reduced to judgmental descriptions of positive symptoms in areas of social, communicational, and functional skills: if at least six symptoms are positive - autism is diagnosed; if less than six are positive with presence of *activities and interests'* symptoms - a pervasive developmental disorder (PDD) is diagnosed; if there are at least two 'social' and one or more 'activities and interests' symptoms without intellectual disability - Asperger` syndrome is diagnosed. If the full criteria for autistic disorder are met and there is no intellectual or cognitive disability, then the individual is diagnosed with highly functioning autism (HFA).

The word 'autism' comes from the Greek term *autos* which means 'self,' in terms of self-isolation, living in own world closed for the "social inventory." Autistic children are often named "old souls," who already "figured out" what adults still have to test over the course of their life-trial. It is hard to suggest whether the scarce verbal, spiritual or metaphysical communications in autistic individuals are the causes or the outcomes of their dense insights. Thus, factors that potentate or remedy the autism are still open for debates.

Sleep is a phenotype. Developmental problems in children, particularly those occurring during the prenatal period, can override or masquerade as genetic influences and contribute in the sleep symptomatic. These problems are especially prominent in children with hyperactivity. When coexisting, behavioral problems alter the sleep pattern in an additive manner.

There is an increased awareness of nocturnal breathing disorders and their complexity in ASD. Over 50% of children with ASD have difficulties in sleep initiation and maintenance,[116] associated with their social skills, communication disturbances, and activity level. [49, 69, 86] Prolonged sleep onset latency, increased daytime sleepiness, parasomnias, bruxism, sleep fragmentation, rapid eye movement abnormality, and obstructive sleep apnea (OSA) associated with the upper airway obstruction, are repeatedly reported in children with classic autism and ASD. [43, 92, 93, 121, 123, 145] A tremendous scholarly resource is mobilized to elucidate why autistic children *"do not breath enough,"* to interpret or at least to describe their *"breathing phobia"* linked to social phobia that creates a havoc for the attached family.

OSA is presented with the prevalence of 1–3% in children, 2–4% of adults, and up to 15% in aging people. [2, 126] It is accompanied by significant daytime cognitive and behavioral deficits that extend beyond the effects of sleepiness. One puzzling aspect of OSA is the difference in behavioral manifestations of prepubertal children versus adults. Adult OSA is associated with the occupational and social failures related to poor planning, disorganization, excessive daytime sleepiness, diminished judgment, rigid thinking, poor motivation, otherwise called *executive dysfunction*, and *affective lability.* [12, 33, 38, 114] Childhood OSA displays a school failure, diminished self-regulation of affective and *arousal state,* [8, 9, 62, 63] an overlay of *hyperactive behaviors*, and *poor impulse control* reminiscent of ADHD [1, 18, 107, 131, 132] that is less evident in adults with OSA. [32, 136]

In all ages, sleep disruption and blood gas abnormalities induce cellular injury of cerebrovascular and cardiovascular systems.[20, 37] This in turn, leads to dysfunction of prefrontal regions of the brain cortex, manifested behaviorally in *executive dysfunction* which markedly affects the functional application of cognitive abilities, resulting in *maladaptive daytime behaviors,*[40, 45, 95] *behavioral inhibition,*[7] poor set-shifting (ability to move from one cognitive or behavioral strategy to another, thinking laterally, being innovative),[65, 115] impaired self-regulation of affect and arousal; [75] short-term working memory (sketch-pad for visual, and phonological loop for verbal information),[106] poor analysis-synthesis (creative thinking, problem solving),[13] and impaired contextual memory (one, that places information into a context of meaningful time-temporal memory, and space-source memory).[106]

The first step of treatment of OSA in adults is the application of *continuous positive airway pressure* (CPAP) via the mask and surgery is used only in selected cases. [5, 64] In contrast, initial treatment of choice for pediatric OSA consists of surgical removal of adenoids and tonsils, with CPAP being reserved for cases in which surgery is contraindicated. Applications of the CPAP during sleep have been reported to improve daytime functioning, however, residual deficits on tests of executive functioning remain particularly evident.[10, 13, 14, 52, 97] Moreover, there is some evidence that in children residual learning deficits may occur long after sleep-disordered breathing has resolved. [62, 63]

Cognitive and adaptive development appears playing a role in frequency of sleep problems from micro and macrostructural viewpoints.[57, 129] Regressive children have significantly less efficient sleep, less total sleep time, prolonged sleep latency, prolonged REM latency, lower cyclic alternating pattern, and more time awake after sleep onset than non-regressive, typically developed children. [76] Others suggest that the IQ is not associated with overall sleep characteristics in children with autism and Asperger's syndrome, however, it has strong associations with night wakening. [104, 144]

Without absolute agreement between studies, findings suggest that children with autism have longer sleep latency, increased stage-1 sleep duration, decreased non-REM sleep, slow-wave sleep (stages 3 and 4), fewer stage 2 EEG sleep spindles, frequent sleep fragmentations, higher density of muscle twitches, and lower sleep efficiency. The objective total sleep time correlates negatively with the *Social and Communication scales* of the *Revised Autism Diagnostic Interview*, and has no correlations with the state anxiety scores of *Spielberger Scale* and cortisol levels. [67, 81, 83, 102, 125] Some psycho educational parameters, such as perception and eye-hand coordination, show significant correlation with sleep parameters: time in bed, sleep latency, stage shifts, first REM latency and wakefulness after sleep onset. *Childhood Autism Rating Scale* (CARS) scores to visual response and non-verbal communication show significant correlation with some tonic sleep parameters, such as sleep period time, wakefulness after sleep onset, and total sleep time. The existence of a sleep pattern in autistic patients is different from that in children with mental retardation and from that in TDP. [22, 28, 36, 49, 110]

Sleep problems are frequent in Angelman syndrome and often severe.[39] Angelman children show higher percentage of wakefulness after sleep onset and sleep onset latency, and reduced REM latency. Higher periodic limb movements index (PLMI), and AHI contribute to cognitive impairment in Angelman children. [90]

Insufficient sleep does not significantly interfere with daytime alertness and sleep problems commonly regress by late childhood, with continuing improvement through adolescence and adulthood. Sleep problems in Angelman syndrome reflect abnormal neuro-developmental functioning presumably involving dysregulation of GABA-mediated inhibitory influences in thalamocortical interactions. Management primarily involves behavioral approaches.[105] Melatonin improves sleep in insomniac patients with Angelman syndrome. [19, 21]

Patients with Asperger's syndrome show decreased sleep time, increased number of shifts into REM sleep from a waking epoch, signs of REM disruption, and increased PLMI. Studies suggest that defective sleep control systems may be associated with clinical picture of Asperger`s syndrome. [61, 68, 103] Sleep macrostructure in children with Lennox-Gastaut syndrome is featured by difficulties in falling asleep, early awakening, and circadian rhythm disorder. Seizures mostly occur during non-REM sleep. [48, 79, 120, 128]

Age of the Rett girls is negatively correlated with night sleep, and positively correlated with day sleep.[109] The Rett syndrome shows markedly impaired sleep/wake patterns, the sleep dysfunction worsens over time and is related with impaired secretion of melatonin.[94] The breathing phenotype is abnormal during sleep and wakefulness; it is extremely complex *(hyperventilation, breath holds, forced and deep breathing and apneutic breathing)* and includes disturbances in cardiorespiratory coupling. This abnormalities are exaggerated during wakefulness and can be worsened by behavioral arousal. [50, 60,72, 87, 88]

Total sleep time in children with Gilles de la Tourette syndrome is controversially being reported as reduced, [73] normal, [34] or longer. [74] Despite unaltered REM sleep children with Tourette syndrome have markedly disturbed sleep with increased arousal phenomena, nocturnal myoclonus syndrome, delta-sleep (slow-wave) reduction, which may be intrinsic to the disorder and might trigger tics and other behavioral problems during daytime. [17, 98, 122] The prevalence of sudden infant death syndrome (SIDS) is Tourette children is 2-5 times higher than that in general population. [133] Severity of Tourette's syndrome during the day positively correlates with number of awakenings and sleep stage changes, and negatively correlates with sleep efficiency. Tic frequency as well as frequency of regular movements is significantly higher in REM than in non-REM sleep. Increased motor activity may be attributable to a state of hyper arousal rather than a disturbed cholinergic system. [56, 139]

RATIONALE

Studies report on low melatonin levels in individuals with ASD, but the underlying cause of this deficit is unknown. [99] Synthesis of melatonin, the key regulator of circadian or seasonal rhythms, and sleep-wake cycle, is encoded by the *ASMT* gene located on the pseudo-autosomal region of sex chromosomes, deleted in several individuals with ASD.[89]

The growing research evidence indicates that sleep disorders, including ideopatic insomnia in children with autism, Angelman, Rett, and Lennox syndromes may relate with an impaired secretion of melatonin as part of the phenotype. [42, 100] The administration of melatonin appears to be a safe treatment of sleep deprivation of ASD children, yet long-term effects of chronic melatonin use in pediatric patients are unknown at this time.[88]

Analyses of the sleep logs disclose a significant treatment effect of melatonin on advancing sleep onset latency, improving total sleep duration, and sleep efficiency.[35] Melatonin is safe with short-term use. [25] Yet, there is no evidence that melatonin is effective in treating secondary sleep disorders. Although melatonin appears to be well-tolerated, its optimal dosage and duration of its administration in autism, Angelman and Rett children, are still debated. [4, 35]

The Mozart effect is believed to be linked with sleep regulation and influences the immune system. [26, 27] The effect varies between the individuals and depends upon the spatial tasks chosen; general intelligence is not affected. Rather more impressively, there is a beneficial effect on some patients with epilepsy.

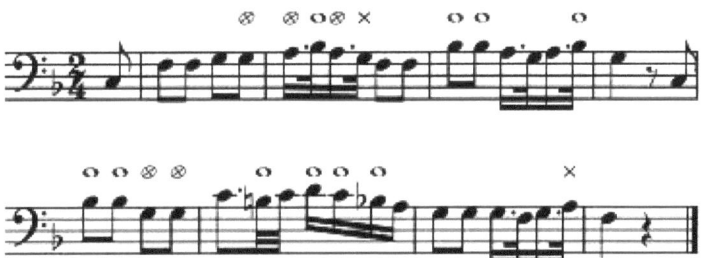

The transforming power of Mozart's music is believed to be linked to its rhythmical and melodic patterns that express humor, joy or sorrow with balancing conviction and mastery. This combination of riveting, never boring properties may reprogram or reset spatial-temporal circuits, improve attention and enhance the thought organization.

Research on the Mozart`s music began in France in late 1950s when Dr. Alfred Tomatis explored auditory stimulation for children with speech and communication disorders. He was the first to introduce the term *"Mozart Effect"* in 1991, in his book *"Pourquoi Mozart."* He advocated alternative medicine solutions for dyslexia, depression, autism and other learning disorders. Since, myriads of studies are focused on the effects of music with high frequencies, especially violin concertos and symphonies, to help children with dyslexia, speech disorders, and autism. By the end of the 20th century it was common knowledge among parents that listening to classical music, especially Mozart, was mandatory in aiding the cognitive development of children.

Why Mozart is special? Neurologist John Hughes at the University of Illinois Medical Center proposes that because Mozart had a habit of repeating certain melodic phrases with slight variation, his melodies tend to repeat patterns every 20-30 seconds, which is about the same length of time as brain-wave patterns and other functions of the central nervous system.

A substanital number of studies suggests on the increase of *mean spatial-temporal IQ scores* after listening Mozart for 10-15 minutes, as measured by various tests derived from the *Stanford—Binet Scale.* [113, 141] Generality of the original positive findings has been criticized on the grounds that any Mozart effect is due to 'enjoyment arousal' occasioned by this particular music and would not take place in the absence of its appreciation.[117] Professor F. Tims (1999) from Michigan State University reports that patients with Alzheimer's Disease who underwent music sessions four times a week increased their level of melatonin, the neurohormone linked with sleep regulation and believed to influence the immune system. This was later confirmed by other studies. [70, 77]

INTENT

An attempt is made to explore and meta-analytically explain the effectiveness of exogenous melatonin in improving sleep in ASD children from the various strata of developmental syndromes. Derived of the data about the Mozart Effect - as an endogenous melatonin stimulator, we intend to inform further research replications on healing threshold of Mozart`s music in sleep problems among children with ASD.

METHODOLOGY

Of the total retrieved 148 articles and book chapters available at PubMed and SCOPUS, studies of level I-IIIA evidence, presenting empirical knowledge on sleep problems (night terror, sleep walking, bed-wetting, sleep-onset anxiety, delayed sleep-phase syndrome, parasomnias, sleep apnea, narcolepsy) in children with ASD were allocated for this meta-assessment.

The data on sleep architecture obtained through sleep diaries, parental reports, actigraphy, and overnight polysomnography of 1,823 ASD children without attention-deficit hyperactivity disorder (ADHD) were compared with the sleep macrostructure of 1,190 typically developed peers. The *efficacy reviews* included randomized controlled trials; the *safety reviews* also included non-randomized studies. Sleep analyses according to the *Rechtschaffen and Kales* procedure were supplemented by counting epochs with short arousal-related movements (≤15 s), thus allowing to calculate correlations between motor activity and sleep parameters.

Children were included in a group defined as having ASD if they scored above the threshold on the *Autism Spectrum Screening Questionnaire* (ASSQ). The sample was inclusive for the age (0-15 years) and diagnosed ASD syndromes: classic autism (Kanner`s), Angelman, Asperger`s, Heller`s, Lennox Gastaut, Rett, and Tourette syndromes. Children with somatic and metabolic problems that contribute in sleep deprivation (hypertrophic cardiopathy, asthma, hypothyroidims, gastroenterocolitis, parasitic infections of skin, others) were excluded from the sample. Mental retardation was not used as a diagnostic criterion.

DIAGNOSTIC CONFIRMATION & DEFINITIONS

Sleep stage/epoch scoring and associated events, arousal analysis, paroxysmal activities, sleep respiration analysis, were defined by the manual of the *American Academy of Sleep Medicine* (AASM, 2007), *American Sleep Disorders Association* (ASDA), and *International Classification of Sleep Disorders:* Diagnostic & Coding Manual (ICSD) criteria.

Rapid eye movement (REM) latency is defined as the period of time in the sleep period from sleep onset to the first appearance of REM sleep.

Sleep efficiency is the ratio of time asleep to the time spent in bed. *Sleep latency* is defined as the time from lights out to sleep onset.

Excessive daytime sleepiness is the subjective report of an increased desire to fall asleep and lack of energy during the day even after an adequate night's sleep.

Apnea is defined as a ≥90% decrease in airflow for ≥10 seconds with preservation of respiratory effort.

Hypopnea is defined as a ≥50% decrease in the airflow for ≥10 seconds, associated with an EEG arousal or an oxygen desaturation of ≥3%.

Obstructive sleep apnea (OSA) is defined by an apnea *index* (AI - apneas per hour of sleep) of ≥1 or an *apnea-hypopnea index* (AHI -number of apneas and hypopneas per hour of sleep) of ≥5.

Nocturnal myoclonus or *periodic limb movements index* (PLMI) is the number of repetitive and highly stereotyped limb movements occurring during one hour sleep.

Arousal index is an abrupt change in the pattern of brain wave activity, as measured by an EEG, that typically represents a shift from deep to light non-REM sleep or from sleep to wakefulness.

Arousal disorder is featured by any of parasomnia (sleepwalking, sleep terrors, and confusing arousals) characterized by atypical arousal from sleep.

The ASD were defined based on criteria developed by the *World Health Organization* (WHO), *Autism Society of America* (ASA), *Mayo Clinic, Diagnostic and Statistical Manual of Mental Illnesses* (DSM), and *American Psychiatric Association* (APsA).

(1) Children were defined in the spectrum of classic Autism ***(Kanner's syndrome)*** for having severe and pervasive impairment in several areas of development, appearing during the first three years of life and impacting development in the areas of social interaction and communication skills *(social phobia, social anxiety, delayed speech, inability to engage in conversation, repetitive movements, motor apraxia, reduced ankle mobility, history of gross motor delay and toe-walking, inflexible routines, preoccupation with abnormal interests or parts/functioning of objects, limited eye contact, inappropriate facial expressions and emotional responses, avoidance of physical contact, others)*. The EEG typical patterns may include: slow wave activity, less alpha, and less inter - and intra hemispheric asymmetry, gamma-band bursts, right-side dominance of the spectral power of *alpha band* at baseline and during the cognitive tasks.

(2) ***Angelman syndrome*** was defined as a genetic disorder that causes developmental disabilities with the onset at 6-12 months, arrested head growth in 2 years, and neurological problems *(difficulty in speaking, balancing and walking, seizures, frequent smiles and outbursts of laughter, hyperactiveness, short attention span, fascination with water, etc)* with the onset at 3-6 years. The EEG shows large amplitude, slow-spike waves.

(3) *Asperger`s syndrome* was defined as pervasive developmental disorder distinguished by a pattern of symptoms characterized by qualitative impairment in social interaction, stereotyped and restricted patterns of behavior, activities and interests, and absence of clinically significant cognitive and speech delay *(intense preoccupation with a narrow subject, one-sided verbosity, restricted prosody, physical clumsiness, circumstantial speech, abrupt transition, marked verbosity, poor hand-writing, poor visual-motor integration, apraxia, odd movements, tandem gait, delayed motor dexterity, limited empathy, reciprocity, social anxiety, repetitive interests and rituals, enhanced perception of small details and patterns, increased sensitivity to sound and light, among others).* The EEG features may include but not limited in: significant attenuation of the *Mu* rhythm when executing an action, and reduced attenuation when observing movement.

(4) Children were defined as having childhood disintegrative disorder (CDD), or **Heller`s syndrome**, if they had shown developmental delays, retarded head growth starting from age of 3 years, and sudden loss of language, social function, and motor skills at the age between 2-10 years *(impaired auditory responsiveness and verbal communication, fearfulness).* The EEG records paroxysmal abnormality associated with temporal cortex and adjacent cortical structures.

(5) *Lennox-Gastaut syndrome (LGS)* was diagnosed in children who had onset of multiple seizure types before age 11 years, with at least one focalized or generalized tonic-axial, myoclonic, atonic or seizure type resulting in falls, and an EEG demonstrating diffuse slow spike-wave complexes (<2.5 Hz), also named as *'petit mal variant.'* Other symptoms included *aggressiveness, antisocial personality, destructive behavior, depression, infantile spasms, hypersexuality, etc.*

(6) *Rett syndrome* was defined as a severe developmental disorder present mostly in girls, manifested with small hands and feet, deceleration of the cranial growth as early as in 5-6 months, physical growth failure, repetitive hand movements, seizures, absence of the verbal skills, gut, scoliosis, constipation, gastroesophageal reflux, poor circulation *(cold, blue extremities),* and typical EEG with the *Theta* rhythm of central region and vicinity.

(7) *Gilles de la Tourette syndrome* was detected for its onset in 7-15 years, characterized by multiple transient and chronic physical (motor) *tics and at least one vocal (phonic) tic, mild speech delay with coprolalia, echolalia, palilalia, chorea, shoulder shrugging, jumping, obsessions, anxiety, depression, self-injurious, attention deficit,* and non-specific EEG architecture with sharp waves and slowing.

MEASURABLE OUTCOMES

The following diagnostic inventories were applied to estimate and measure the outcomes:

Abberant Behavior Checklist (ABC),

Abstract Objective Rett syndrome (RTT),

Autism Behavior Checklist (ABC),

Autism Diagnostic Observation Schedule (ADOS),

Behavioral Evaluation of Disorders of Sleep (BEDS),

Choice Assessment Scale (CAS),

Gilliam Asperger's Disorder Scale (GADS),

International Classification of Sleep Disorders-Second Edition (ICSD-2),

Nocturnal Polysomnography (NPSG),

Revised Autism Diagnosis Interview (ADI-R),

Tourrette`s Syndrome Severity Scale (TSSS),

The Yale Global Tic Severity Scale (YGTSS),

Vinelad Adaptive Scale,

as well as the parental reports in

Children's *Sleep Habits Questionnaire* (CSHQ), and

Pittsburgh *Sleep Quality Index* (PSQI).

The empirical data was supplied by the nuclear ribonucleoprotein polypeptide N (SNRPN) assay, and also, by the established chromosomal and gene abnormalities.

- **Primary outcome measures:** sleep latency, REM latency, apnea, parasomnias, sleep efficiency in seven syndromes stratified for unmedicated children with ASD, and their age-matched controls.

- **Secondary outcome measures:** total sleep time (measured by actigraphy), decreased number of awakenings (measured by actigraphy), periodic limb movement index, apnea/hypopnea index, in melatonin-induced children.

DATA EXTRACTION & ANALYSIS

The descriptive statistics were carried out by means of *one-way analysis of variance* (ANOVA) in continuous data, *Kruskal-Wallis* ANOVA for ranked ordinal data, and *Likelihood Ratio Chi-square* (X^2) where the data were categorical. *Intraclass correlations* (ICC) between the groups were assessed to avoid spurious correlations. Factors with *Chronbach's alpha* above 0.400 were considered as comparative. Varied factor-loading thresholds were examined with the optimal threshold yielding correlations greater than 0.40.

For binary variables relative risk (RR) and its 95% confidence interval (CI) were computed on an intention to treat bias. Continuous data were presented by weighed mean difference statistic, with a 95% CI and alpha level below 0.05.

For the multivariate models generalized estimating equations were used with the queue of Pearson's arrival. Gender and age of children were included in all models to adjust for the study design. Final multivariate linear regression models were fitted to determine whether sleep factors derived from exploratory factor analysis and total amount of sleep by parental reports were associated with diagnoses and delays in cognitive or adaptive development. Computations were held with the help of ASSISTAT (version 7.6 ß, 2011) and KeyPlot (version 2.0 ß 15, 2001) programs.

RESULTS

The sleep battery of 1,823 children and teens aged 0-15 years and diagnosed with autism (n = 656; 36%), Angelman (n = 166; 9.1%), Asperger`s ($n$ = 277; 15.2%), Heller`s (n = 293; 16.07%), Lennox-Gastaut (n = 98; 5.37%), Rett (n = 184; 10.1%), and Gilles de la Tourette syndromes (n = 149; 8.17%) were extracted from 64 studies of levelI-IIIA evidence and compared to their age-match, typically developed peers (n = 1,190). Sixty two percent (62%) of children were males. *Table 1* presents general parameters of the ASD and the linked sleep symptomatic:

Table 1:   General Characteristics of Autism and ASD

As seen from *Table 1,* the ASDs have complex and diverse interplay in terms of its onset, occurrence, sex ratio, genetic coding, degree of developmental delay, and prognosis. Fairly similar in behavioral expressions, the spectrum syndromes manifest in a wide variety of combinations and specifics in sleep macrostructure.

Children with classic autism are more likely to be disoriented after waking, with increased daytime sleepiness (narcolepsy), tendency to OSA associated with upper airway obstructions. Angelman children are featured with greater rates of somnambulism (prolonged wakefulness after sleep onset), reduced REM sleep, higher

Syndromes

Differential properties	Autism (Kanner's)	Angelman	Asperger's	Heller's	Lennox-Gastaut	Rett	Gilles de la Tourette
Lifetime incidence	20-50 /10,000	0.4-1/10,000	4.1-7.1 / 1,000	1.6-6.4 / 100,000	2/100,000	1/10,000-23,000	10/1,000
Age-adjusted incidence in preschool children	5.5/100,000	1/12,000-20,000	3-6/1,000	6-7 /1,000	0.26/1,000	0.22-1/10,000	1-10 /1,000
Lifetime prevalence	0.01 - 0.5%	0.01%	0.02 - 0.13%	0.71%	0.03%	0.01%	1-2%
One-time prevalence among children with ASD	65.27%	1.3-4.8%	0.58%	0.20%	4% among childhood epilepsy	3.47%	6.50%
Male/Female ratio	3.9- 4.3 / 1	1 / 2	1.6-5. / 1	4 / 1	Equal	Females, only	1.8- 4 / 1
Causality	Prenatal influences on dopamine activity; maternal psychosocial stress, maternal fever, maternal STD, maternal use of certain medications, urban birth, fetal hypoxia, MMR vaccination; Mercury induced	Genetic: maternally inherited	Antenatal exposure to teratogens; Abnormal migration of embryonic cells	Antenatal infections; teratogens, toxins; thimerosal-containing vaccines	Tuberous sclerosis, perinatal asphyxia, severe head brain injury, encephalitis, meningitis, lesions of frontal lobe, inherited degenerative or metabolic conditions, maternal toxoplasmosis, rubella	Genetic. X-linked disorder; males die soon after birth	Post-streptococcal autoimmune disorder, hypothyroidism, encephalitis
Genetic defects	Fragile X syndrome, Chromosome 22 Trisomy; 20/22 Translocation; 22q11.2 deletion;	Chromosome 15q11-q13 deletion, microdeletion, uniparental	There are rare descriptions of Chromosome 17p breakpoints	Yet unknown	Chromosome 9 ring 4 abnormalities	Sporadic mutations of the gene on X chromosome encoding	Yet unknown

	some data on 22q11.2 duplication	disomy, or an imprinting center defect; Absence of functional copy of maternal UBE3A gene				Mecp2 protein	
Age at the onset	3 years	2-3 years	3 years	2 years	2-8 years	6-18 months	6-15 years
Drug-naïve dopamine content	Increased	"Happy puppet"	Slightly increased	Lower	Generally decreased	Decreased or normal	Increased
Arrested head growth:	None declared (often have macrocephalus)	2 years	None declared (often have macrocephalus)	3 years	None declared	5-6 months	None declared
Developmental delay	Moderate to significant	Severe	Mild	Severe	Mild and progressing	Severe	Mild
Speech	Echolocation, delayed speech without communicative gesturing, inability to engage in conversation	Absent of severe impairment	Mild disturbance: poor prosody, circumstantial speech, abrupt transition; marked verbosity	Severe impairment, dramatic loss	Reduced verbal fluency, poor communication	Absent or severe impairment	Coprolalia, echolalia, palilalia
Social withdrawal	Present, Phobia	None declared	Phobia, anxiety	Present	Present	Present	May be present
Movement / Balance disorders	Repetitive movements, hypotonia, motor apraxia, reduced ankle mobility, history of gross motor delay and toe-walking	Ataxic gait, tremulous movement of hands, seizures	Poor hand-writing, poor visual-motor integration, apraxia, clumsiness, odd movements, tandem gait, delayed motor dexterity	Seizures	Daily multiple Blitz Nick Salaam seizures, localized or generalized axial, axorhizomelic, tonic, myoclonic, atonic seazures with falls, dropp attacks	Stereotypic hand wringing, gait dyspraxia, seizures, oral-motor dysfunction, loss of purposeful use of hands	Multiple motor tics and at least one utterance (phonic tic), chorea, shoulder shrugging, jumping
Behavioral phenotype	Mood disorders, social anxiety; lack of pretend play, inflexible routines, preoccupation with abnormal interests or	Frequent laughter, easily excitable and happy, hand flapping, hyperactive, short attention span	Limited empathy, social anxiety, repetitive interests and rituals, enhanced perception of small details and	Impaired auditory responsiveness and verbal communication, fearfulness	Aggressiveness, antisocial personality, destructive behavior, depression	Screaming episodes, ataxia, poor social interactions, panic attack.	Obsessionality, anxiety, depression, self-injurious, attention deficit

	parts/functioning of objects, limited eye contact, inappropriate facial expressions and emotional responses, avoidance of physical contact	fascination with water	patterns, increased sensitivity to sound and light		infantile spasms, hypersexuality	avoidance of eye contact, bruxism	No specifics
Concurrent clinical, metabolic manifestations	Gastro-intestinal dysfunction, food intolerance	Strabismus, increased sensitivity to heat, hypopigmented skin and hair	Coeliac disease, Food intolerance	Tuberous sclerosis (benign brain tumor), lipid storage disease (excess fat in nervous system), sclerosing panencephalities, may lose bladder and bowel control	Are related to side effects of anticonvulsants: respiratory insufficiency, asthma, aplastic anemia, gastroenteritis, periodontitis, gingival swelling, nonketonal hyperglycinemia	Gut, scoliosis, constipation, gastroesophageal reflux, poor circulation, cold, blue extremities.	
Cognitive impairment	Moderate to significant with paradoxic enhanced memory	Present	Absent or mild	Dementia	May be present	Dementia	Absent
Sleep architecture	Prolonged sleep onset latency, increased daytime sleepiness, parasomnias, sleep fragmentation, REM abnormality, obstructive sleep apnea associated with upper airway obstruction	Sleep apnea that improves with age, frequent nocturnal awakenings, excessive daytime sleepiness, oxygen desaturation in REM sleep, increased periodic leg movement	Alexithymia, difficulty in falling asleep, frequent nocturnal awakenings, early morning awakenings	None specified	Difficulty in falling asleep and early awakening, circadian rhythm disorder. Seizures mostly occur during non-REM sleep	Sleep disturbance during regression, normal breathing during sleep, neurotrophic respiratory disorder, disorganized breathing patterns while	Nocturnal myoclonus syndrome, arousal disorder, delta-sleep (slow-wave) reduction

index of PLM, sleep fragmentations, and reduced total sleep. Children with Asperger`s and Lennox syndromes exhibit frequent patterns of early morning awakenings, and nocturnal terror. Tourette`s children have disturbed sleep quality with increased arousal phenomena, which both may be intrinsic to the disorder and might trigger tics and other behavioral problems during daytime. Their breathing

							awake.
EEG features	Slow wave activity, less alpha, and less inter- and intrahemispheric asymmetry, gamma-band bursts, right-side dominance of the spectral power of the alpha band at baseline and during cognitive tasks	Large amplitude slow-spike waves	Significant attenuation of the Mu rhythm when executing an action, and reduced attenuation when observing movement	Paroxysmal abnormality associated with temporal cortex and adjacent cortical structures	Diffuse slow spike-wave complexes, 'petit mal variant'	Theta rhythm of central region and vicinity	Usually uneventful but may present sharp waves and slowing
Life expectancy	Normal	Normal	Normal	Normal	3-7% mortality	40-50 year life-expectancy	Normal
Treatment	Targeted treatment of Fragile X syndrome, gamma interferon inhibitor, IL-1 beta, IL-6, IL-12, IL-18, and TNF-alpha inhibitors, IL-10, self-help skills development, special education with early intervention	Treatment of seizures, OT	Early intervention-education, social skill development, OT, sedation	Behavioral and speech therapy	Symptom directed: anticonvulsants, anesthetics, steroids, immunoglobulins	Treatment of constipation, GERD, OT, weight loss, foliate, L-dopa, beta-blockers, SSRI	Neurologists, cholinolytic comatose therapy, surgical-stimulation of the anterior internal capsule
Cure	None	None	Curable	None	None	None	Yet none
Works cited:	6, 15, 16, 41, 76, 84, 91, 96, 111, 119, 127	29, 89, 100, 107, 108, 143	15, 30, 47, 58, 134	55, 76, 79, 84, 138	11, 51, 59, 70, 78, 120, 128, 137	23, 31, 53, 63, 72, 82, 135, 142, 146	3, 34, 44, 48, 54, 112, 120, 122, 130, 140, 147, 148

patterns worsen while awake. When coexisting, Tourette syndrome and behavioral problems alter the sleep pattern in an additive manner.

The EEG profiles autistic children with slow wave activity, right-side dominance of the spectral power of *alpha-band*, and *gamma-band* bursts. Angelmen children show large amplitude slow-spike waves, Asperger`s children - *Mu* rhythm changes per action and movements; Heller`s children-paroxysmal abnormality associated with temporal cortex; Lennox children- diffuse slow spike-wave complexes, Rett girls - *Theta rhythm* of central region, and Tourette syndrome presents sharp waves and slowing. Although, agreement among objective studies is not absolute, these data suggest increased nighttime activity, reduced rapid eye movement sleep, and significant daytime somnolence in unmedicated children with ASD when compared to controls.

The subjective and objective data on sleep architecture, utilized for meta-assessment, were obtained through sleep diaries, parental reports, actigraphy, and overnight polysomnography. Twenty-nine out of the total reviewed studies, utilized subjective sleep-reports, eleven were actigraphic studies, and twenty were overnight polysomnographic sleep studies (six of which also included *Multiple Sleep Latency Tests*). *Table 2* illustrates the extracted data on sleep architecture in unmedicated children with seven ASD (page 93):

Overall prevalence of sleep disorders is twice higher in autism (RR 2.1), Lennox (RR 2.14), and Rett syndromes (RR 2.5) than that in age-matched TDP ($p < .02$). Total sleep time is notably reduced in Lennox-Gastaut children (OR 1.4; $p < .02$). A longer sleep onset latency is presented in children with autism (OR 2.58), Asperger`s (OR 2.7), Rett (OR 3.4), and Tourette syndromes (2.8) ($p < .03$). Angelman kids have the lowest arterial oxygenation counts (RR 0.7). *Apnea-hypopnea index* is twice higher in children with classic autism (2.1), and Angelman (2.0) syndrome, and thrice higher in children with Asperger`s (2.87) and Heller`s (3.0) syndromes ($p < .02$). Nocturnal

Table 2: *Battery of sleep architecture in unmedicated children and teenagers with autism and ASD*

Sleep Architecture	Autism	Angelman	Asperger's	Heller's	Lennox	Rett	Tourette	Control
Sample size	656	166	277	293	98	184	149	1190
Mean age (years)	8.16 (±3.9)	12.4 (±9.6)	8.7 (±4.8)	9.2 (±6.6)	7.5 (±4.4)	9.5 (±6.8)	9.5 (±2.5)	8.9 (±4.4)
Age range (years)	3-15	2-15	5-10	3-16	3-16	1-13	5-12	4-16
Male/Female ratio	6.7/1	1/1.2	7/1	4.1/1	1.15/1	Females only	4.3/1	7.4/1
Intelligence quotient (IQ) mean	98.4 (8.6)	62.5 (17.5)	102.7 (11.4)	50.5 (13.5)	69.7 (14.3)	52 (26.8)	105.3 (10.2)	103.3 (8.5)
Prevalence of sleep disorders (%)	63.15	54	59.9	50.8	62.5	73.6	47.8	29.16
Total sleep time (h)	7.71 (0.67)	7.6 (0.96)	7.98 (0.61)	8.4 (0.93)	6.5 (0.86)	7.5 (0.33)	8.8 (1.12)	9.39 (1.1)
Sleep onset latency (min)	32.7 6.93	24.8 (7.84)	33 (6.38)	24.11 (4.31)	13.8 (2.49)	42.1 (11.8)	34.2 (9.3)	12.3 (2.13)
REM latency (%)	12.75	26.3	24.9	16.6	33.9	28.1	17.1	16.68
AHI (per hour)	4.3 (2.6)	4.24 (1.9)	5.7 (1.7)	6.2 (0.9)	3.18 (2.6)	3.03 (2.2)	2.76 (2.2)	2.04 (1.45)
Arterial oxygen saturation index (%)	87.7	75.7	87	89.2	82.5	89.9	88	96.3
PLMI (per hour)	4.3 (2.6)	3.96 (2.0)	5.58 (3.9)	12.6 (8.2)	13.05 (9.1)	9.16 (4.7)	6.62 (2.19)	2.82 (1.9)
Diurnal bruxism (%)	21	20.9	19.7	48	38.2	21.5	20.8	14.8
Central apnea (%)	46.8	49.1	25	25	44.6	57	20	10.43
Total Arousal Index (per/hour)	16.04 (9.5)	12.3 (4.56)	3.25 (0.9)	17.1 (8.7)	14.8 (7.0)	7 (3.0)	19.1 (6.7)	6.5 (3.52)
Sleep efficiency (%)	89.96	90.57	86.9	90	92.8	78.57	84.5	96.4
Daytime naps (%)	31	21.2	31.2	34	64.5	24.5	61.5	22.35

Student T- test (p), or Pearson test for trend (X^2 P) < 0.05; 95% CI , ns = not significant

Works allocated for the meta-analysis: 3, 4, 9-11, 16, 18, 20, 21, 23-25, 28, 34-37, 39, 42, 43, 48-50, 52, 56, 57, 60-64, 67-69, 74, 76, 81, 83, 85, 87, 88, 92-95, 100, 102-105, 108, 110, 106, 116, 118, 122, 123, 126, 129, 131, 136, 139, 144

bruxism and the mean index of periodic limb movement are more evident in Heller`s (RR 3.2; 4.4), Lennox (RR 2.6; 4.6), and Rett (RR 1.5; 3.2) children ($\chi^2$=5.097). However, increased arousal index (OR 2.4; $p < .03$), and decreased REM latency (OR 0.7; $p <.05$) profile only children with autism, Heller`s, and Tourette syndromes.

Table 3: Correlation Matrix per Syndrome

Syndromes	IQ	SOL	AHI	PLMI	CA	AI	SE
Autism	ns	ns	SOL * β= .9256	ns	ns	ns	ns
Angelman	ns	SE * β = .8894	ns	ns	AI * β = -.8832	CA -* β = -.8832	SOL * β = .8894
Asperger`s	ns	ns	ns	ns	ns	ns	ns
Heller`s	ns	AI * β = -.8914	ns	CA ** β = -.9972	PLMI** β = -.9972	SOL * β = -.8914	
Lennox	ns	ns	ns	ns	ns	ns	ns
Rett	ns	AI ** β = .9999	SE* β = -.9356	ns	ns	SE* β = -.8918	AHI, AI* β = -.9356
Tourette	SE ** β = -.9650	CA * β = -.9017	ns	ns	AI * β = -.9273	SOL ** β = .9965	IQ ** β = -.9650
Control	SE ** β = -.9710	ns	ns	ns	IQ ** β = .9625	ns	CA ** β = -.9697
Index	IQ- intelligence quotient; SOL-sleep onset latency; AHI-apnea/hypopnea index; PLMI-periodic limb movement index; CA-central apnea; AI-arousal index; SE-sleep efficiency						

Note: The correlation coefficient β is presented only, when significant.
The vacant cells present non-significant (ns) correlations (p >= .05)
** Significant at level of 1% of probability (p < .01).
 * Significant at level of 5% of probability (.01 =< p < .05)
 Positive correlations;   Negative Correlations.

Table 3 presents the matrix of Pearson correlations between developmental disorders and sleep symptomatic. As established, in Tourette`s children exclusively, cognitive scores are negatively related to sleep onset parameters (- 0.9017, p < .05). In autistic children the prolonged sleep onset latency correlates with increased apnea/hypopnea index (0.9256, p<.05).  In  children with Angelman, Heller`s and

Tourette`s syndromes, sleep fragmentations are less associated with respiratory stimuli (-.08832, - 0.9972, and - 0. 9273, correspondingly, p < .01). In Rett girls the arousal index related to respiratory stimuli is more suitable to show the degree of sleep fragment (-0.9356; p <.05). The affected sleep efficiency in Rett children is related to frequent arousals and obstructive apnea. In Asperger`s children central apnea and daytime sleep duration are negatively correlated with age (-0.8957; - 0.9226; correspondingly, p<.05).

Findings suggest that sleep-maintenance insomnia and inefficient sleep in ASD children may have moderate associations with polysomnography-defined central apnea, arousal index, but not with periodic limb movement index and cognitive development. These results require confirmation but suggest that clinical assessment of central apnea and arousal index may be helpful but not yet definitive. Statistical corrections for overall agreement and specificity of this findings show 87% weighed-agreement and 26% adjusted specificity.

Data on melatonin efficacy and safety were collected from treatment studies. A total of 146 children with baseline sleep abnormalities and with confirmed diagnoses of Autism (n=107), Asperger`s (n=20), Angelman (n=8) and Rett (n=11) syndromes aged between between 2-15 years, underwent a 4-week melatonin treatment in a double-blind, placebo-controlled, crossover protocol that employed a 1-week washout between treatment trials. Melatonin doses ranged from 2.5 to 7.5 mg at nocturnal bedtime, based on the individual BMI. The efficacy was measured through parental diary records of lights off time, sleep onset, night wakes, wake-up time, epileptic seizures (if applicable), and polysomnographic records. In case of inefficacy, melatonin dose could be titrated up to 9 mg the following 2 weeks at increments of 3 mg/week, unless the child was unable to tolerate it. The analysis of all the sleep logs disclosed a significant treatment effect of melatonin on sleep latency (p=0.025).

After initiation of melatonin, 25% of parents of autistic children no longer reported sleep concerns at follow-up visits. Improved sleep was reported in 60% children, and continued sleep problems were reported in 13% of children. In 2.8% of children mild side-effects were detected, including morning sleepiness and increased enuresis. In children with autism melatonin significantly decreased sleep-onset latency to 19.1 ± 5.3 minutes ($p < 0.05$) during the first 3 weeks of treatment. It improved total sleep time and sleep efficiency at the 4th week. In Asperger`s children melatonin reduced sleep latency to 21.4 ± 2.7 minutes ($p < .05$). However, no difference in the number of awakenings was noted.

In Angelman children with ideopatic insomnia, melatonin significantly advanced sleep onset by 28 ± 1.8 minutes ($p < .05$), decreased sleep latency by 32 ± 5.6 minutes ($p < .05$), increased total sleep time by 56 ± 9.8 minutes ($p < .03$), reduced the number of nights with wakes from 3.1 to 1.6 nights a week, and increased endogenous salivary melatonin levels. After 4 weeks of open treatment however, there was in some patients a tendency to a reduction in therapeutic gain. In children whom the treatment lost its effect, melatonin levels had become extremely high, whereby the normal 24h melatonin rhythm was lost. Findings indicate that the melatonin metabolism in Angelman children is disturbed as is part of the phenotype.

In Rett girls, melatonin treatment appeared to poorly influence the seizure frequency. Exogenous melatonin dramatically improved the sleep-wake cycle, but early morning awakenings occurred occasionally. When treatment was stopped, the sleep disorders recurred and re-administration of 3 mg melatonin was effective. The effect was maintained over 2 years without any adverse effects. These findings suggests that sleep disorders in patients with Rett syndrome may relate with an impaired secretion of melatonin.

Based on this review we conclude that melatonin is safe with the short term use. Also, yet there is no evidence that melatonin is effective in treating secondary sleep disorders. Controlled trials to determine efficacy appear warranted.

DISCUSSIONS

Sleep is indeed, a complex phenotype. Developmental problems in children, particularly those occurring during the prenatal period, can override or masquerade as genetic influences, and contribute in this phenotype. Problems with sleep onset and maintenance are also common in typically developing children.

It is estimated that up to 1/3 of toddlers and preschoolers have nighttime waking. These problems may be especially prominent in children with hyperactivity and oppositionality. When coexisting, these behavioral problems alter the sleep pattern in an additive manner. It has been suggested that neurodevelopmental disorders predispose children to sleep–wake rhythm disturbances, perhaps because of the difficulties in perception and interpreting of cues needed for synchronizing sleep with the environment. This decreased synchronization is often accompanied by the abnormal melatonin secretion.

We tried to determine the developmental components associated with sleep disorders stratified for seven autistic spectrum syndromes, and to explore the safety and efficacy of melatonin administration in those disorders. Sixty-four studies of level I-IIIA evidence from the samples of 1,823 autism spectrum children and their 1,190 typically developing peers (TDP) where allocated for the meta-assessment. The sleep battery components (total sleep time, sleep onset latency, REM latency, arousals, periodic limb movements, apneas, bruxism, sleep efficiency, other parasomnias) derived from subjective (ADOS, ADI-R, ABC, BEDS, CSHQ, ICSD-2, RTT, PSQI inventories), and objective measures (polysomnography, actigraphy) were modeled as measurable outcomes. Thirty six percent (36%) of children were diagnosed with Autism, 9.1 % with Angelman, 15.2% with Asperger`s, 16.1% with  Heller`s, 5.37% with Lennox-Gastaut, 10.1% with Rett, and 8.17% with Gilles de la Tourette syndromes. Sixty- two percent of subjects were boys.

Prevalence of sleep disorders was twice higher in Autism, Lennox, and Rett syndromes. The most commonly reported sleep problems (difficulty falling asleep, restless sleep, central apneas, and sleep fragmentations) likely reflected problems with the sleep–wake cycle, confirming findings of previous studies. [144] A longer sleep onset latency was present in children with autism, Asperger`s, Rett, and Tourette`s syndromes. Apnea-hypopnea index was 2-3-fold higher in children with classic autism, Angelman, Asperger`s, and Heller`s syndromes. The lowest sleep efficiency was found in Rett girls.

No age related differences were noted in reported and measured sleep problems other than central apnea and daytime sleep duration in Asperger`s children. In contrary to previous studies [57, 76, 116, 129] we did not find that sleep symptomatic, especially parasomnias, were related to children's cognitive and intellectual deficits, except of Tourette children, whose cognitive scores were negatively related to sleep onset parameters (β = - 0.9017). This statement is consistent with the previous studies suggesting that sleep problems occur among children with autism at all IQ levels and are similar in nature. [104] Our findings support a relatively low incidence of most parasomnias among children with Autism, Asperger`s and Rett syndrome; however paradoxically, the Rett girls are found to be the least satisfied from sleep.

Growing evidence indicates that sleep disorders in children with autism, Angelman, and Rett syndromes may relate with impaired secretion of melatonin. Administration of the exogenous melatonin in children with classic Autism, Angelman, Asperger`s and Rett syndromes appear to improve the sleep-wake cycle (60%), total sleep time, sleep efficiency, and advance sleep-onset latency at the 3rd-4th weeks of treatment. However, no difference in the number of awakenings is noted. Overall, melatonin is safe with short term use. Yet, there is no evidence that melatonin is effective in treating secondary sleep disorders. Although melatonin appears to be well-tolerated, its optimal dosage and duration of administration in autism, Angelman and Rett children, are still discussed.

In search for the alternative or naturalistic approaches, we found that the Mozart effect is linked with sleep regulation and increases the endogenous melatonin secretion. While, existing empirical data on Mozart`s effect on sleep onset and efficacy are limited in studies of TDP, current study informs replications of further research on Mozart`s effect on sleep macrostructure in children with autism and its spectrum disorders.

Limitations: This study did not address some issues, such as severity and duration of sleep problems, nor it was designed to distinguish between the sleep problems associated with comorbid conditions other than mental retardation. Further, the meta-assessment was based on both objective (actigraphic and polysomnographic) and subjective (provider or parental reports) measures. Next, it did not delineate the degree of visual or auditory impairment in those reporting these problems. Finally, it did not measure the impact of sleep deprivation on the academic performance of children.

CONCLUSIONS

Fairly different in their expressions, prevalence of sleep onset disorders, sleep fragmentations, impaired nocturnal breathing, and reduced sleep efficiency is twice higher in children with autism, Rett, Tourette`s, Angelman, and Heller`s syndromes. Age does not relate to sleep problems other than central apnea (-0.8957) and daytime sleep duration (0.9226) in Asperger`s children. Our findings suggest that sleep symptomatic, especially parasomnias, are not related to children's cognitive and intellectual deficits, except of Tourette`s children whose cognitive scores are negatively related to sleep onset parameters (- 0.9017). Sleep-maintenance insomnia, and inefficient sleep have moderate associations with polysomnographically-defined central apnea, arousal index having acceptable sensitivity (87%) but low specificity (26%). The administration of melatonin appears to improve sleep-wake cycle (60%), and advance sleep-onset latency, but does not impact on arousal index. Although melatonin is well-tolerated, its optimal dosage and duration are not established yet.

IMPLICATIONS FOR RESEARCH

Further research is required to examine comorbid conditions in pediatric sleep symptomatology. Based on the evidence that sleep deprivation in ASD children is related with melatonin deficits, and that the Mozart effect may stimulate endogenous melatonin production, this study informs extensions of further studies in Mozart's effect on treatment of sleep disorders among children with autism and ASD.

ACKNOWLEDGMENTS

Conflict of Interest: None declared.

Consent of Subjects: This was a systematic review, intact of human subject, tissues, organs, biological fluids, or animal models.

Setting: This was the solo study of the author.

Dedication: This study is dedicated to *Mayo Clinic Foundation.*

INDEX OF TERMS

Rapid eye movement	REM	4, 11, 21
Relative risk	RR	15, 21, 23
Sleep onset latency	SOL	23
Stanford—Binet Scale	SBS	9
Sudden infant death syndrome	SIDS	7
Tourrette`s syndrome severity scale	TSSS	14
The Yale Global Tic Severity Scale	YGTSS	14
Typically developed peers	TDP	10, 21, 26, 28
Vinelad Adaptive Scale	VAS	15

WORKS REVIEWED AND CITED:

(1) **Ali NJ, Pitson DJ. Stradling JR (1996).** Sleep disordered breathing: effects of adeno-tonsillectomy on behavior and psychological functioning. *European Journal of Pediatrics,* 155: 56–62

(2) **Ali NJ, Stradling JR (2000).** Epidemiology and natural history of snoring and sleep-disordered breathing. *Marcel Dekker, New York,* 555–574.

(3) **Allen RP, Singer HS, Brown JE, Salam MM (1992).** Sleep disorders in Tourette syndrome: A primary or unrelated problem? *Pediatric Neurology;* 8(4):275-280

(4) **Andersen IM, Kaczmarska J, McGrew SG, Malow BA (2008).** Melatonin for insomnia in children with autism spectrum disorders. *Journal of Child Neurology;*23(5):482-5

(5) **Arens R (2000).** Obstructive sleep apnea in childhood. *Marcel Dekker, New York;* 575–600

(6) **Barbaresi WJ, Katusic SK, Colligan RC, Weaver AL, Jacobsen SJ (2005).** The incidence of autism in Olmsted County, Minnesota, 1976-1997. *Archives of Pediatrics & Adolescent Medicine;* 159(1).

(7) **Barkley RA (1997).** Behavioral inhibition, sustained attention, and executive functions: constructing a unifying theory of ADHD. *Psychology Bulletin;* 121: 65–94.

(8) **Barkley RA (2000).** Genetics of childhood disorders. *Journal of the American Academy of Child and Adolescent Psychiatry;* 39: 1064–1068.

(9) **Bates JE, Viken RJ, Alexander DB, Stockton L(2003).** Sleep and adjustment in preschool children: sleep diary reports by mothers relate to behavior reports by teachers.

Child Development; 73(1):62-75

(10)**Bearpark H, Grunstein R, Touyz S, Channon L, Sullivan CE (1987).** Cognitive and psychological dysfunction in sleep apnea before and after treatment with CPAP. *Sleep Research;* 16: 303.

(11)**Beaumanoir A, Warren B (1992).** The Lennox-Gastaut Syndrome: Epileptic Syndromes in Infancy, Childhood, and Adolescence; *John Libbey & Eurotext Ltd;* 125-148

(12)**Beebe DW, Gozal D (2002).** Obstructive sleep apnea and the prefrontal cortex: towards a comprehensive model linking nocturnal upper airway obstruction to daytime cognitive and behavioral deficits. *Journal of Sleep Research;* 11(1):1-16

(13)**Bedard M A (1991).** Obstructive sleep apnea syndrome: pathogenesis of neuropsychological deficits. *Journal of Clinical and Experimental Neuropsychology;* 13: 950–964.

(14)**Bedard MA, Montplaisir J, Malo J, Richer F, Rouleau I (1993).** Persistent neuropsychological deficits and vigilance impairment in sleep apnea syndrome after treatment with continuous positive airway pressure (CPAP). *Journal of Clinical and Experimental Neuropsychology;* 15: 330-341.

(15)**Bernier R, Dawson G, Webb S, et al (2007).** EEG *mu* rhythm and imitation impairments in individuals with autism spectrum disorder. *Brain and Cognition;* 64(3):228-237

(16)**Berry-Kravis E, Knox A, Hervey C (2011).** Targeted treatments for fragile X syndrome. *The Journal of Neurodevelopmental Disorders;* 3(3):193-210

(17)**Bonnier C, Nassogne M-C, Evrard Ph (1999).** Ketanserin treatment of Tourette's syndrome in children. *American Journal of Psychiatry;* 156:1122A-1123

(18)**Bower CM, Gungor A (2000).** Pediatric obstructive sleep apnea syndrome. *Otoloaryngologic Clinics of North America;* 33: 49-75.

(19)**Braam W, Didden R, Smits MG, Curfs LM (2008).** Melatonin for chronic insomnia in Angelman syndrome: a randomized placebo-controlled trial. *Journal of Child Neurology;*23(6):649-54.

(20)**Bradley TD, Floras JS (2000).** Sleep apnea: Implications for cardiovascular and cerebrovascular disease. *Dekker, New York*

(21)**Bruni O, Ferri R, D'Agostino G, Miano S, Roccella M, Elia M (2004).** Sleep disturbances in Angelman syndrome: a questionnaire study. *Brain Development;* 26(4):233-40

(22)**Buckley AW, Rodriguez AJ, Jennison K, Buckley J, Thurm A, Sato S, Swedo S (2010).** Rapid eye movement sleep percentage in children with autism compared with children with developmental delay and typical development. *Archives of Pediatric and Adolescent Medicine;* 164(11):1032-7

(23)**Burd L, Vesley B, Martsolf JT, Kerbeshian J (2005).** Prevalence study of Rett syndrome in North Dakota children. *American Journal of Medical Genetics;* 38(4):565-568

(24)**Bokkala S, Nepalinga K, Pinninti N, Carvalho CS, Valencia I, Legido A, Sanjeev V (2008)**. Correlates of periodic limb movements of sleep in the pediatric population. *Pediatric Neurology;* 39(1):33-39

(25) **Buscemi N, Vandermeer B, Hooton N, et al. (2006).** Efficacy and safety of exogenous melatonin for secondary sleep disorders and sleep disorders accompanying sleep restriction: meta-analysis. *BMJ;* 332:385

(26) **Campbell D (1997).** The Mozart Effect. *Avon Books;* New York

(27) **Campbell D (2000).** The Mozart Effect for children. Harper Collins*:* New York

(28) **de Carvalho LB, do Prado MB, de Almeida MM, et al (2004).** Cognitive dysfunction in children with sleep disorders. *Arquivos de Neuro-Psiquiatria;* 62:2

(29) **Cassidy SB, Dykens E, Williams CA (2000).** Prader-Willi and Angelman syndromes: Sister imprinted disorders. *American Journal of Medical Genetics;* 97(2):136-146

(30) **Chakrabarti S, Fombonne E (2005).** Pervasive developmental disorders in preschool children: confirmation of high prevalence. *The American Journal of Psychiatry;* 162:1133-1141

(31) **Chao HT, Chen H, Samaco RC, et al (2010).** Dysfunction in GABA signaling mediates autism-like stereotypes and Rett syndrome phenotypes.. *Nature;* 468(7321):263-9

(32) **Chervin RD (1997).** Symptoms of sleep disorders, inattention, and hyperactivity in children. *Sleep;* 20: 1185–1192

(33) **Cheshire K (1992).** Factors impairing daytime performance in patients with sleep apnea/hypopnea syndrome. *Archives of Int. Med;* 152: 538–541

(34) **Cohrs S, Rasch T, Altmeyer S, et al (2001).** Decreased sleep quality and increased sleep related movements in patients with Tourette's syndrome. *Journal of Neurological and Neurosurg Psychiatry;* 70(2): 192–197

(35) **Coppola G, Iervolino G, Mastrosimone M, La Torre G, Ruiu F, Pascotto A. (2004).** Melatonin in wake–sleep disorders in children, adolescents and young adults with mental retardation with or without epilepsy: a double-blind, cross-over, placebo-controlled trial. *Brain & Development;* 26(6):373-376

(36) **Couturier JL, Speechley KN, Steele M, Norman R, Stringer B, Nicolson R (2005).** Parental perception of sleep problems in children of normal intelligence with pervasive developmental disorders: prevalence, severity, and pattern. *Child & Adolescent Psychiatry;* 4(8):815-822

(37) **Culebras A (1999).** Sleep disorders and neurological disease. *Marcel-Dekker Inc,* New York

(38) **Day R (1999).** The behavioral morbidity of obstructive sleep apnea. *Progress in Cardiovascular Diseases;* 41: 341–354

(39) **Didden R, Korzilius H, Smits MG, Curfs LM (2004).** Sleep problems in individuals with Angelman syndrome. *American Journal of Mental Retardation;* 109(4):275-84

(40) **Diomedi M (1998).** Cerebral hemodynamic changes in sleep apnea syndrome and effect of continuous positive airway pressure treatment. *Neurology;* 51: 1051–1056

(41) **Dissanayake C, Bui QM, Huggins R, Loesch DZ (2006).** Growth in stature and head circumference in high-functioning autism and Asperger's disorder during the first 3 years of life. *Development and Psychopathology;* 18:381-393

(42) **Dodge NN, Wilson GA (2001).** Melatonin for treatment of sleep disorders in children with developmental disabilities. *Journal of Child Neurology;* 16(8):581-584

(43) **Doo S, Wing YK (2006).** Sleep problems of children with pervasive developmental disorders: correlation with parental stress. *Developmental Medicine & Child Neurology;* 48(8):650-5

(44) **Drake ME Jr, Hietter SA, Padamadan H, Bogner JE (1991).** Computerized EEG frequency analysis in Gilles de la Tourette syndrome. *Clinical EEG;* 22(4):250-3.

(45) **Dyken ME (1996)**. Investigating the relationship between stroke and obstructive sleep apnea. *Stroke;* 27: 401–407

(46) **Eapen V, Fox-Hiley P, Banerjee S, Robertson M (2004).** Clinical features and associated psychopathology in a Tourette syndrome cohort. *Acta Neurologica Scandinavica;* 109(4):255-60.

(47) **Ehlers S, Gillberg C (1993).** The Epidemiology of Asperger Syndrome. *Journal of Child Psychology and Psychiatry;* 34(8):1327-1350

(48) **Eisensehr I, Parrino L, Noachtar S, Smerieri A, Terzano MG (2001).** Sleep in Lennox–Gastaut syndrome: the role oft the cyclic alternating pattern (CAP) in the gate control of clinical seizures and generalized polyspikes. *Epilepsy Research;* 46(3):241-250

(49) **Elia M, Ferri R, Musumeci SA, Del Gracco S, et al (2000).** Sleep in subjects with autistic disorder: a neurophysiological and psychological study. *Brain and Development;* 22(2):88-92

(50) **Ellaway C, Peat J, Leonard H (2001).** Sleep dysfunction in Rett syndrome: lack of age related decrease in sleep duration. *Brain Development;* 23 Suppl 1:S101-3.

(51) **Engel J, Pedley TA, Aicardi J (2008).** Epilepsy: A comprehensive textbook, 2nd edition. *Lippincott Williams & Wilkins,* Vol.3

(52) **Feuerstein C, Naegelé B, Pépin JL, Lévy P (1997).** Frontal lobe-related cognitive functions in patients with sleep apnea syndrome before and after treatment. *Acta Neurologica Belgia;* 97: 96-107.

(53) **FitzGerald PM, Jankovic J, Percy AK (1990).** Rett syndrome and associated movement disorders. *Movement Disorders;* 5(3):195-202

(54) **Flaherty AW, Williams ZM, Ramin A, et al (2005).** Deep brain stimulation of the anterior internal capsule for the treatment of Tourette Syndrome: Technical case report. *Neurosurgery;* 57(4):E403

(55) **Fombonne E (2002).** Prevalence of childhood disintegrative disorder. *Autism;* 6(2):149-157

(56) **Freeman RD, Fast DK, Burd L, Kerbeshian J, Robertson MM, Sandor P(2007).** An international perspective on Tourette syndrome: selected findings from 3500 individuals in 22 countries. *Developmental Medicine and Child Neurology;* 42(7):436-447

(57) **Giannotti F, Cortesi F, Cerquiglini A, Vagnoni C, Valente D (2010).** Sleep in children with autism with and without autistic regression. *Journal of Sleep Research;* 20(2):338-347

(58) **Gillberg C, Souza L (2002).** Head circumference in autism, Asperger`s syndrome, and ADHD: a comparative study. *Developmental Medicine and Child Neurology;* 44(5):296-300

(59) **Glauser T, Diego MA (2002).** Introduction. Lennox-Gastaut Syndrome. *eMedicine.com, Inc.*

(60) **Glaze DG, Frost JD, Zoghbi HY, Percy AK (1987).** Rett's syndrome: Characterization of respiratory patterns and sleep. *Annals of Neurology;* 21(4):377-382

(61) **Godbout R, Bergeron C, Limoges E, Stip E, Mottron L (2000).** A laboratory study of sleep in Asperger`s syndrome. *Neuro Report;* 11:1

(62) **Gozal D, Wang M, Pope DW (2001).** Objective sleepiness measures in pediatric obstructive sleep apnea. *Pediatrics;* 108: 693-697.

(63) **Gozal D, Pope D (2001).** Snoring during early childhood and academic performance at ages thirteen to fourteen years. *Pediatrics;* 107:1394-1399

(64) **Guilleminault C, Lee JH (2005).** Pediatric obstructive sleep apnea syndrome. *Archives of Pediatric and Adolescent Medicine;* 159:775-785

(65) **Harrison Y, Horne JA, Rothwell AL (2000).** Prefrontal neuropsychological effects of sleep deprivation in young adults: A model for healthy aging? *Sleep;* 23: 1067-1073.

(66) **Harvey A, Andersen AO, March M (1999).** Learn with the classics. Using music to study smart at any Age. *LIND Institute.*

(67) **Hering E, Epstein R, Elroy S, Iancu DR, Zelnik N(1999).** Sleep patterns in autistic children. *Journal of Autism and Developmental Disorders;* 29(2):143-147

(68) **Hiie A (2006).** Asperger's syndrome and high-functioning autism in school-age children : the children's sleep and behavior, and aspects of their parents' well-being. *Karolinska Instituten* (Doctoral Thesis)

(69) **Hoffman CD, Sweeney DP, Gilliam GE, et al (2005).** Sleep problems and symptomatology in children with autism. *A Journal of Hammill Institute on Disabilities;* 20(4):194-200

(70) **Horowitz S (2004).** Music Therapy: Notes from research and clinical practice. *Alternative and Complementary Therapies;*10(5): 251-256.

(71) **Ieshima A, Takeshita K (1987).** Chromosome abnormalities and epileptic seizures. *Japanese Journal of Human Genetics;* 33: 49–60

(72) **Katz DM, Dutschmann M, Ramirez J-M, Hilaire G (2009).** Breathing disorders in Rett syndrome: Progressive neurochemical dysfunction in the respiratory network after birth. *Respiratory Physiology and biology;* 168(1-2): 101–108

(73) **Kirov R, Kinkelbur J, Banaschewski J, Rothenberger A (2007).** Sleep patterns in children with attention-deficit/hyperactivity disorder, tic disorder, and comorbidity. *Journal of Child Psychology and Psychiatry;* 48(6):561-570

(74) **Kostanecka-Endress T, Banaschewski T, Kinkelbur J, et al (2003).** Disturbed sleep in children with Tourette syndrome: A polysomnographic study. *Journal of Psychosomatic Research;* 55(1):23-29

(75) **Kotterba S, Rasche K, Widdig W, et al (1998).** Neuropsychological investigations and event-related potentials in obstructive sleep apnea syndrome before and during CPAP-therapy. *Journal of Neurol. Science;* 159: 45-50.

(76) **Krakowiak P, Goodlin B (2008).** Sleep problems in children with autism spectrum disorders, developmental delays, and typical development: a population-based study. *Journal of Sleep Research;* 17(2):197-206

(77) **Kumar AM, Tims F, Cruess DG, et al (1999).** Music therapy increases serum melatonin levels in patients with Alzheimer's disease. *Alternative Therapies in Health and Medicine;* 5(6):49-57

(78) **Kurita H, Koyama T, Osada H (2005).** Comparison of childhood disintegrative disorder and disintegrative psychosis not diagnosed as childhood disintegrative disorder. *Psychiatry and Clinical Neurosciences;* 59(2):200-5

(79) **Laakso ML, Leinonen L, Hätönen T, Alila A, Heiskala H (1993).** Melatonin, cortisol and body temperature rhythms in Lennox-Gastaut patients with or without circadian rhythm sleep disorders. Journal *of Neurology;* 240(7); 410-416

(80) **Lazoff T, Zhong L, Piperni T, Fombonne E (2010).** Prevalence of pervasive developmental disorders among children at the English Montreal School Board. *Canadian Journal of Psychiatry;* 55(11):715-20

(81) **Limoges É, Mottron L, Bolduc C, Berthiaume C, Godbout R (2005).** Atypical sleep architecture and the autism phenotype. *Brain*; 128, 1049–1061

(82) **Lioy DT, Wu WW, Bissonnette JM (2011).** Autonomic dysfunction with mutations in the gene that encodes methyl-CpG-binding protein 2: Insights into Rett syndrome. *Autonomic Neuroscience: basic and clinical;* 161(1-2):55-62

(83) **Liu X, Hubbard JA, Fabes RA, Adam JB (2006).** Sleep disturbances and correlates of children with autism spectrum disorders. *Child Psychiatry & Human Development;* 37(2):179-191

(84) **Lushchekina EA, Podreznaia ED, Lushchekin VS, Strelets VB (2010).** Comparative EEG study in normal and autistic children. *Zh Vyssh Nerv Deiat Im I P Pavlova*;60(6):657-66

(85) **Malhotra S (2002).** Childhood disintegrative disorder. *European Child & Adolescent Psychiatry;* 11(3):108-114

(86) **Malow BA, McGrew SG, Harvey M, Henderson LM, Stone WL (2006).** Impact of treating sleep apnea in a child with autism spectrum disorder. *Pediatric Neurology;* 34(4):325-328

(87) **Marcus CL, Carroll JL, McColley SA, et al (1994).** Polysomnographic characteristics of patients with Rett syndrome. *The Journal of Pediatrics;* 125(2):218-224

(88) **McArthur AJ, Budden SS (1998).** Sleep dysfunction in Rett syndrome: a trial of exogenous melatonin treatment. *Developmental Medicine & Child Neurology;* 40(3):186-192

(89) **Melke J, Botros HG, Chaste P, et al (2008).** Abnormal melatonin synthesis in autism spectrum disorders. *Molecular Psychiatry;* 13: 90–98

(90) **Miano S, Bruni O, Elia M, Musumeci SA, Verrillo E, Ferri R (2005).** Sleep breathing and periodic leg movement pattern in Angelman Syndrome: A polysomnographic study. *Clinical Neuropsychology;* 116(11): 2685-92

(91) **Ming X, Brimacombe M, Wagner GC (2007).** Prevalence of motor impairment in autism spectrum disorders. *Brain & Development;* 29(9):565-70

(92) **Ming X, Walters AS (2009).** Autism spectrum disorders, attention deficit/hyperactivity disorder, and sleep disorders. *Current Opinion in Pulmonary Medicine;* 15(6):578-584

(93) **Ming Y, Ye-Ming S, Nachajon R, Brimacombe M, Walters AS (2009).** Prevalence of parasomnia in autistic children with sleep disorders. *Clinical Medicine Insights;* 3:1-10

(94) **Miyamoto A, Oki J, Takahashi S, Okuno A (1999).** Serum melatonin kinetics and long-term melatonin treatment for sleep disorders in Rett syndrome. *Brain and Development;* 21(1):59-62

(95) **Mohsenin V, Culebras A (2001).** Sleep-related breathing disorders and risk of stroke editorial comment: Balancing sleep and breathing. *Stroke; 3*2;1271-1278

(96) **Mukaddes NM, Heguner S (2007).** Autistic disorder and 22q11.2 duplication. *World Journal of Developmental Psychiatry;* 8(2):127-130

(97) **Naëgelé B, Thouvard V, Pépin JL**, et al **(1995).** Deficits of cognitive executive functions in patients with sleep apnea syndrome. *Sleep;,* 18: 43-52.

(98) **Nee LE, Caine ED, Polinsky RJ, Eldridge R, Ebert MH (1980).** Gilles de la Tourette syndrome: Clinical and family study of 50 cases. *Annals of Neurology;* 7(1):41-49

(99) **Nir I, Meir D, Zilber N, Knobler H, et al (1993).** Brief report: Circadian melatonin, thyroid-stimulating hormone, prolactin, and cortisol levels in serum of young adults with autism. *Journal of Autism and Developmental Disorders;* 25 (6): 641-654

(100) **O'Callaghan FJ, Clarke AA, Hancock E, et al (2007).** Use of melatonin to treat sleep disorders in tuberous sclerosis. *Developmental Medicine & Child Neurology;* 41(2):123-126

(101) **Oiglane-Shlik E, Talvik T, Žordania R, et al (2006).** Prevalence of Angelman Syndrome and Prader–Willi Syndrome in Estonian Children. *American Journal of Medical Genetics;* 140A:1936–1943

(102) **Øyane NM, Bjørvatn B (2005).** Sleep disturbances in adolescents and young adults with autism and Asperger's syndrome. *Autism;* 9(1):83-94

(103) **Paavonen EJ, Vehkalahti K, Vanhala R, Aronen ET, von Wendt L (2008).** Sleep in children with Asperger syndrome. *Journal of Autism and Developmental Disorders;*38(1):41-51

(104) **Patzold LM, Richdale AL, Tonge BJ (2002).** An investigation into sleep characteristics of children with autism and Asperger's Disorder. *Journal of Pediatric and Child Health;* 34(6):528-533

(105) **Pelc K, Cheron G, Boyd SG, Dan B (2008).** Are there distinctive sleep problems in Angelman syndrome? *Sleep Medicine:* 9(4):434-41.

(106) **Pennington BF (1997).** Dimensions of executive functions in normal and abnormal development. In: Krasnegor GR. Development of the Prefrontal Cortex: Evolution, Neurobiology, and Behavior. Paul H. *Brookes Publishing, Baltimore,:* 265-281.

(107) **Perkin RM, Downey R, MacQuarrie J (1999).** Sleep-disordered breathing in infants and children. *Respiratory Care Clinics of North America;* 5: 395-426.

(108) **Petersen MB, Brøndum-Nielsen K, Hansen LK, Wulff K (2005).** Clinical, cytogenetic, and molecular diagnosis of Angelman syndrome: Estimated prevalence rate in a Danish county. *American Journal of Medical Genetics;* 60(3):261-262

(109) **Piazza CC, Fisher W, Kiesewetter K, Bowman L, Moser H (1990).** Aberrant sleep patterns in children with the Rett syndrome. *Brain and Development;* 12(5):488-93

(110) **Polimeni MA, Richdale AL, Francis AJ (2005).** A survey of sleep problems in autism, Asperger's disorder and typically developing children. *Journal of Intellectually Disabled Children;* 49(Pt 4):260-8.

(111) **Previc FH (2007).** Prenatal influences on brain dopamine and their relevance to the rising incidence of autism. *Medical hypothesis;* 68(1): 46-60

(112) **Pushkov V (1986).** Treatment of Tourette syndrome. *Zh Nevropatol Psikhiatr Im S S Korsakova;* 86(10):1476-9

(113) **Rauscher FH, Shaw GL, Ky KN (1995).** Listening to Mozart enhances spatial-temporal reasoning: toward a neurophysiological basis. Neurosci Lett;185: 44-7

(114) **Redline S, Strohl KP (1999).** Recognition and consequences of obstructive sleep apnea hypopnea syndrome. *Otolaryngologic Clinics of North America;* 32: 304-331

(115) **Redline S, Strauss ME, Adams N, et al (1997).** Neuropsychological function in mild sleep-disordered breathing. *Sleep;* 20: 160-167.

(116) **Richdale AL (1999).** Sleep problems in autism: prevalence, cause, and intervention. *Developmental Medicine and Child Neurology;* 41(1):60-6

(117) **Rideout BE, Dougherty S, Wernert L (1998).** Effect of music on spatial performance: a test of generality. Percept Motor Skills; 86: 512-14.

(118) **Rutter M (2005).** Incidence of autism spectrum disorders: Changes over time and their meaning. *Acta Paediatrica;* 94(1): 2-15

(119) **Rutter M, Taylor EA (2002).** Child and adolescent psychiatry. *Blackwell Science, Inc,* 4th edition

(120) **Saleh TA, Stephen L (2008).** Lennox-Gastaut syndrome, review of the literature and a case report. *Head & Face Medicine;* 4:9

(121) **Saletu A, Parapatics S, Anderer P, Matejka M, Saletu B (2009).** Controlled clinical, polysomnographic and psychometric studies on differences between sleep bruxers and controls and acute effects of clonazepam as compared with placebo. *European Archives of Psychiatry & Clinical Neuroscience;* 260(2): 163-174

(122) **Sandyk R, Bamford CR, Iacono RP (1987).** Sleep disorders in Tourette's syndrome. *International Journal Of Neuroscience;* 37(1-2): 59-65.

(123) **Serra-Negra JM, Paiva SM, Seabra AP, et al (2010).** Prevalence of sleep bruxism in a group of Brazilian schoolchildren. *European Archives of Pediatric Dentistry;* 11(4):192-5.

(124) **Singer HS, Szymanski S, Giuliano G, et al(2002).** Elevated intrasynaptic dopamine release in Tourette's Syndrome measured by PET. *The American Journal of Psychiatry;* 159:1329-1336

(125) **Sivertsen B, Posserud MB, Gillberg C, Lundervold AJ, Hysing M (2011).** Sleep problems in children with Autism spectrum problems: A longitudinal population-based study. *Autism;* 16(2):139-50

(126) **Skatrud JB, Dempsey JA (1983).** Interaction of sleep state and chemical stimuli in

sustaining rhythmic ventilation. *Journal of Applied Physiology: Respiratory, Environmental & Exercise Physiology;* 55(3):813-22.

(127) **Skurkovich B (2006).** Treatment of autism. WO/Patent/002058

(128) **Slapal R, Zouhar A (1989).** Therapeutic effect of dopaminergic substances in drug-resistant Lennox-Gastaut syndrome. *Cesk Neurol Neurochir.;* ;52(1):32-5.

(129) **Souders MC, Mason TB, Valladares O, et al (2009).** Sleep behaviors and sleep quality in children with autism spectrum disorders. Sleep; 32(12):1566-78.

(130) **Staedt J, Stoppe G, Kögler A, et al (1995).** Noctural myoclonus syndrome (periodic movements in sleep) related to central dopamine D2-receptor alteration. *European Archives of Psychiatry and Clinical Neuroscience;* 245(1):8-10

(131) **Stores G (1999).** Children's sleep disorders: modern approaches, developmental effects, and children at special risk. *Developmental Medicine & Child Neurology;* 41: 568-573

(132) **Stradling JR, Stradling JR, Thomas G, Warley AR, Williams P, Freeland A (1990).** Effect of adenotonsillectomy on nocturnal hypoxaemia, sleep disturbance, and symptoms in snoring children. *The Lancet;* 335: 249-253.

(133) **Sverd J (1993).** Is Tourette syndrome a cause of sudden infant death syndrome and childhood obstructive sleep apnea? *American Journal of Medical Genetics;* 46(5)

(134) **Tentler D, Johannesson T, Johansson M, et al (2003).** A candidate region for Asperger syndrome defined by two 17p breakpoints. *European Journal of Human Genetics;* 11:189–195.

(135) **Terai K, Munesue T, Hiratani M, Jiang ZY, Jibiki I, Yamaguchi N (1995).** The prevalence of Rett syndrome in Fukui prefecture. *Brain & Development;* 17(2):153-4

(136) **Thiedke CC (2001).** Sleep disorders and sleep problems in childhood. *American Family Physician;* 63(2):277-285

(137) **Trevathan E, Murphy CC, Yeargin-Allsopp M (1997).** Prevalence and descriptive epidemiology of Lennox-Gastaut syndrome among Atlanta children. **Epilepsy**,;38(12):1283-8.

(138) **Unal O, Ozcan O, Oner O, Akcakin M, Aysev A, Deda G (2009).** EEG and MRI findings and their relation with intellectual disability in pervasive developmental disorders. *World Journal of Pediatrics;* 5(3):196-200

(139) **Voderholzer V, Müller N, Haag C, Riemann D, Straube A (1997).** Periodic limb movements during sleep are a frequent finding in patients with Gilles de la Tourette's syndrome. *Journal of Neurology;* 8:521-526

(140) **Volkmar FR, Leckman JF, Detlor J,et al (1984).** EEG abnormalities in Tourette's syndrome. *The Journal of the American Academy of Child Psychiatry;* 23(3):352-3

(141) **Wago H, Kasahara S (2004).** Music therapy, a future alternative intervention against diseases. *Advances in Experimental Medicine and Biology;* 546:265-78.

(142) **Wenk GL (1996).** Rett syndrome: evidence for normal dopaminergic function. *Neuropediatrics;* 27(5):256-9

(143) **Williams CA (2005).** Neurological aspects of the Angelman syndrome. *Brain and Development;* 27: 88-94

(144)   **Williams PG, Sears LL, Allard A (2004).** Sleep problems in children with autism. *Journal of Sleep Research;* 13:265-268

(145)   **Whiteford L, Fleming P, Henderson AJ (2004).** Who should have a sleep study for sleep related breathing disorders? *Archives of Disability in Children;* 89:851–855

(146)   **Wong VC, Li SY (2007).** Rett Syndrome: Prevalence among Chinese and a comparison of MECP2 mutations of classic Rett Syndrome with other neurodevelopmental disorders. *Journal of Child Neurology;* 22(12): 1397-1400

(147)   **Yang J, Li GL, Lü BQ (2002).** Genetic features of EEG abnormality in children with Tourette syndrome. *Hunan Yi Ke Da Xue Xue Bao;*27(3):273-4.

(148)   **Zafeiriou DI, Ververi A, Vargiami E (2007)**. Childhood autism and associated comorbidities. *Brain & Development;* 29 (5): 257–72